See the website:

Stay current on the newest methods for getting in shape and regular instructions on improving your surfing.

Copyright © 2021

All rights reserved.

If you would like to email me markap12@gmail.com

If you would like surf lessons, look for Mark's Surf Instruction in Oceanside, CA.

Other Books:

Creating Your Own Happiness*

The Good Life Plan*

The Surfers Life*

Surf Instructions: Beginner to Advanced*

The Surfing Guide

The Surf Course: 30 page audio book

*Available on Amazon

Table of Contents

Intro

Surfing is more about functional age than chronological. We see seniors enjoying all types of recreation in active lifestyles. The key is to get your body ready to be active or improve your fitness to engage in anything you want.

Surfing is a great goal for building fitness. It is a full body exercise that needs muscle, flexibility, and stamina. It is a peak recreation for full body engagement. Many fitness routines can build parts of the body or improve some of the surfing requirements.

Swimming is another full body engagement that is not only complete in itself, but is a great stamina and strength builder for surfing. Biking is a great recreation for leg strength and stamina. Riding a road bike also requires some upper body strength to stay suspended above the handlebars.

Activities that promote flexibility support surfing progress. Being stretched or flexible is helpful in any activity of everyday life. Flexibility prevents injury and can give you the confidence to begin new activities. There are great exercises to build flexibility.

Nutrition is important for any athlete or non-athlete. Everyone needs nutrients to sustain metabolic processes and optimize our physical attributes. A healthy nutritional practice becomes spiritual as we take pride in caring for out bodies.

Surfing is a spiritual experience as we connect with the ocean and Mother Nature. We hold the ocean in awe for its power and beauty. We develop a spiritual connection because we feel so great mixing with its elements and blocking out all other thoughts.

Chapter One

The Fun of Getting Fit

Getting started is usually the biggest obstacle. For one thing, the mind tries to sabotage all good efforts. It tells us that any good new practices are not good for us and will cause us too much pain or discomfort.

Years ago, I went through a four-year process of losing 50 pounds. I was motivated to get back to my high school weight. I was already working out several days a week, but it became obvious my nutrition program was causing me to gain weight.

In the process, I became a witness to what my mind was telling me. It was always against new healthier nutrition ideas and against any new strenuous exercise in which I wanted to engage.

I would listen to what it said and then proceed anyway, thanking it for its input. Sometimes I would engage in new exercises to show my mind it was wrong. On days when it told me I was tired, I considered the message. Then I rationally considered whether the previous day's rest had not been sufficient. Then I would proceed just to show my mind it was wrong.

After a while, the mind flips and becomes our best supporter. It starts to protest bad foods and lazy days when we don't stick to our routine. It becomes an "app" like on our cell phone to support our goals.

Once we are engaged and seeing results, we become more enthused. Who doesn't like to achieve? We start to develop discipline. This may be the most useful characteristic we ever develop.

When you see people who are active, you often find they say it is who they are. When I was running 60 miles a week, I defined myself as a runner. People who bike or climb mountains often mention their activity first when they tell you who they are.

Fitness, health, and nutrition become defining lifestyle practices. They start connecting us with Nature because everything we are doing is good for us and the way Nature intended us to live. Compare us to animals and we find that a healthy lifestyle runs parallel to what God's creatures already do.

Chapter Two

Discipline Becomes Our Greatest Friend

I revere discipline. It makes everything possible. Achievers will add focus, determination, persistence, faith, and lots of other descriptive behaviors and beliefs. Discipline is the will to stay the course.

Discipline is the characteristic that makes us move forward on days we don't want to. If I have started walking or running each morning and on one day, my mind says let's rest today, discipline will have us putting on our shoes when we don't feel like it. Of course, don't ignore real body signs that say rest is needed. Just don't fall prey to a mind that wants you to stop.

Often in the past when I decided to surf in the morning, my mind would say "its so cold and so much work". I realized that each time I had this thought, but put on my wetsuit and went into the water, I was happy I did. The reward of being in the water made me appreciate moving forward and not becoming a victim of a mind that wanted me to be weak.

A mind will bring out the whiny child in us. But, mom, I don't want to. Mom is not there for us to use as a foil now. She has turned us loose. We are our own person and must deal with real life scenarios. Getting fit is for the strong side of us that says we were born to be champions.

Chapter Three

The Importance of Having Purpose

One of the more important aspects of a quality lifestyle as a senior is still feeling purposeful. I mentioned to a friend that I was again writing books and said I was as happy about wanting to write as I was about finishing my books.

I had mentioned that for a while after writing everyday for years, I no longer felt ambitious about writing books or posts. He said you are resting. Having enthusiasm for activities makes life more exciting and fulfilling.

Children and grandchildren are exciting, but its fun to have your own enthusiasm and interests to bring to the table. Being fit so you always feel well is a giant plus for your lifestyle as a senior.

There is a joke about you know you are old when you meet your friends at the pharmacy instead of at the night clubs. It is common place for us seniors to go to the pharmacy often, but we can balance that with exercise and great nutrition.

The goal of wanting to be fit or learning to surf or climbing a mountain are all excellent for motivating new behaviors. The enthusiasm for accomplishing something to be proud of stimulates additional positive behaviors. It can flip us from being mostly negative to mostly positive.

Spiritualists say each day we should feel gratitude, joy, peace, and love. When I meditate each morning, I make these four words part of a prayer. I like to add romance and prosperity. Why not, we're not dead yet. As a writer and surf instructor of 11 years, I like to add fitness as another identity factor to who I am. When surf season slows down, I become a road biker. You can't have too many interests.

Chapter Four

The Spirituality of Surfing

Surfing is a connecting device. If you want to feel connected to Nature, the ocean, and your body, surfing is the best. We know that surfing is physically demanding, so after learning to surf you find that being in better fitness would make surfing more fun and progress more likely.

Now you are considering what makes a body better. We become part of the phenomena that animals don't have to think about. They don't have the luxury of refrigerators or Netflix. They have to look for food everyday and normally have to move to find it. Like early man.

Once we were foragers and hunters. The one advantage man had over all game is he could run them down until they were tired. Hard to believe we could outrun antelopes, but early man could run longer. The advantage of the antelope over the lion is they are both about the same speed, but the antelope can run longer.

When we enter the ocean, we are immediately in awe of the ocean's power and our vulnerability. Surfers that ride giant waves know they could die. Unless they get pinned down underwater, most advanced surfers are prepared for the challenge. They know they have to bring their best game.

Knowing you could always be better is part of the fun. Working to be better both physically and mentally is the challenge. The brain thrives and grows with challenge. The opposite is sameness and atrophy. We are designed to grow until we die.

Bringing your best to the ocean challenge can make surfing exciting every day. Did you win? Did the ocean win? What could you work on to make the next session better? How are you and the ocean getting along?

Feeling connected to the ocean is being connected to Nature. We start to feel all is one. This is the highest spiritual concept. It would mean we see ourselves as one with all things in the Universe and also with mankind. We might stop seeing man's differences and recognizing the similarities.

People that visit Oceanside for surf lessons often say they enjoy how surfers are chill. When you are content in your environment and feel you have found your truth or many truths, your need to find more becomes diminished. The materialistic world stops holding the same allure.

Chapter Five

Risk as a Source of Inspiration

Entrepreneurs live and thrive on risk. We could say anyone pushing the envelope to where they have never been before enjoys risk. Pushing the envelope to where man has never been before is another level many live for. Why climb Everest, go to Mars, beat the 4-minute mile, do a million pushups?

It is human nature to grow. Growth is a requirement of our brain and body or it begins to atrophy. There is no middle ground. Pursuing boundaries is a healthy endeavor. The brain has plasticity, so it can grow until we die. The body's genome can sense whether we are still hunting for food, so to speak, or have quit and are ready to start the dying process.

Risk stimulates healthy chemicals. Serotonin, dopamine, adrenaline, and norepinephrine are just a few hormones and neurotransmitters that get excited when we are on an adventure. Seeking the unknown has always been part of man's nature. Think about how exciting it is to plan an adventure vacation.

Contemplating better fitness is exciting if you can take the first step. Progressively building is an adventure that never has to stop. At every summit, a new summit comes into view.

The master of "flow" Steven Kotler, describes in his book *The Rise of Superman* how extreme athletes get into a state in which their body and mind take over the action and they ride as witnesses to an exhilarating experience of achievement.

I like another author's description of what Kotler's book stands for:

*At its core, this is a book about profound possibility; about what is actually possible for our species; about where—if anywhere—our limits lie. In this groundbreaking book, New York Times–bestselling author **Steven Kotler** decodes the mystery of ultimate human performance.*

Flow can be experienced in lots of activities. Writers, musicians, artists, chefs, hobbyists, and surgeons all describe the state of engaging in activities in which they have competence and pushing the envelope just a little.

We can seek risk at any age. It might awaken us from the stupor or malaise that we have allowed to encompass our spirit. Ambition is a spark that can begin any adventure. If I want to become a renown writer or influence how other people live, I have to begin with the first sentence.

Learning to surf has risks. Most of the risks are not insurmountable. Famous waterman Laird Hamilton has surfed a 100-foot wave and each year at Navarre, Portugal, big wave surfers are on 90' beasts. Most everyone has the capability of learning to surf. It may take some work to get into the proper surf shape to execute properly. Everyone starts at the bottom and works their way up. At the bottom, it is pretty-safe.

As a surf instructor, I encounter a lot of students from children to adults who have not been exercising. They have a difficult time, but still have fun. They also learn that if they want to continue and improve, they might have to start engaging in some physical exercise.

When we think of the change necessary to accomplish a goal, we are contemplating risk. The risk is mostly self-reflection. What if we fail? This is the stopper for most people before they begin. They might have a preconceived notion they can't change or that change is not worthwhile.

One of my young students recently asked me after the dryland portion of a lesson and before we went in the water, "what if I fail"? I was so flabbergasted at the question I asked him to repeat it. "It's ok", I said. I asked another young boy why he seemed to be afraid riding on the surfboard and gave him several options. He jumped on fear of failure. Why is this built into our nature?

Chapter Six

The Beauty of Will Power

All the best intentions are smoke without the willpower to make them come true. We get the spark of an idea, dream, goal, or innovation. Then we create the plan. Discipline keeps us on the plan. Will power overcomes adversity. Will power is the long term driver for success.

Will power is the tactic we utilize to listen to the mind's effort to sabotage our good efforts and decide that our goal is more important than the comfort the mind suggests instead. When I have wanted to add laps to my runs on the beach sand, my mind would say it wasn't a good idea. I thought, I have to teach the mind again who is boss. After that, when I turned the corner for another lap, my mind would just say here we go again.

Health coaches and personal trainers work with clients from the moment they may inquire about improving themselves. The process moves from intentions to a plan to action. Then comes maintenance. In this stage, the client is adhering to the routines and enjoying progress.

Coaches are looking for the step where clients become self-monitoring and engage in the activities without having to be coached or encouraged. At this step the coach can be a guide.

The stage where coaches earn their keep is in relapse. This is often an incident where the client did not follow the plan. They lapsed back into previous habits in which they felt comfortable. Most eager clients that start on a program of improvement relapse after a year.

What happens? The dream dies. The client loses the inspiration of achieving their dream and their old ways look comforting. "It was so much fun when I just ate whatever I wanted." "I have lost 25 pounds, that's enough, I deserve some relief." "This weight program or aerobic fitness is so tiring. I need to rest."

These are all mind tricks. The mind wins. In his book *Resilience*, Navy Seal and Rhodes Scholar, Eric Greiten says Navy Seal bootcamp is the greatest experience you never want to repeat. Most entrants don't complete it. At some point, their minds and bodies say I can't take it anymore. We may all have a point where we draw the line. Finding that line is the quest.

People have saved themselves from the most trying circumstances. We might face physical or emotional challenges. Some say God doesn't give us more than we can handle. Is that true? In many daily events, people find a way to get through more than we should expect them to handle. They become superhuman. Yet, they are just expressing that which we are all capable of.

There is a line at which all great challenges will test our own personal capabilities and willpower. Maybe willpower is a capability. At a point when we are tired, what is the voice that says push on?

When I was in the process years ago of losing 50 pounds, I was at a stage where I was eating raw and exercising hard. I ran a set of stairs that had 40 steps to the beach on a regular basis. One day, my mind said I was too tired to run that day. I thought, I just rested yesterday, that is a lie. I normally ran the steps 20 to 40 times and had once run them 60 times. This day, I ran them 80 times. That took a few hours. Afterward, with pride, I said Ok mind. I guess I am boss and don't do that again.

Of course, the mind does it every day. Who is the boss? You want a piece of chocolate cake and you are on a program to lose weight. The mind drives you insane with desire. You don't think you can take it another moment without indulging. Or, you want to write a book and day after day the mind helps you procrastinate. I have found that once I start writing a book, it just starts to flow and I no longer have to worry about stalling.

Willpower helps us focus. What do you want to achieve? What do you have to do first? What do you have to do next? Let's measure our progress and see if we are on the right path. If we hit a wall, guru, Anthony Hopkins says its time for a new strategy. We don't give up, we create a new path.

Chapter Seven

Beginning the Path to Fitness

What does fitness mean? What does it mean to you? Most people associate fitness with a lean look and the capability to enjoy a fun exercise or recreation. It includes confidence that an exercise or recreation can be completed and not result in injury.

Surfing fitness would make you feel you could surf as long as you want and tackle challenges you desire successfully. We always want to come out of the water without being injured. Tackling bigger challenges is part of surfing just like video gaming. Practice improves performance.

Like making a movie, the backup crew is crucial. An actor looks good because there is a good script, director, editor and other specialists. Surfers are successful because they prepare.

I get lots of surf students who have not exercised. They underestimate the demands of surfing. They learn quickly. The first thing they notice is their lack of flexibility. The beginner surfing pop up I teach requires putting a foot flat on the surfboard under your butt and standing up on that leg. If you can't put the foot flat due to lack of flexibility, it is hard to stand up properly.

Pushing your body up off the surfboard is also important. Without some upper body strength, this simple task becomes difficult. Most lives do not include utilizing upper body strength. We walk, but we rarely lift. We hardly ever stretch. Most activities do not require cardiovascular development.

What about diet? It is easy to see what is happening to physiques in most Western countries. We continuously consume more calories than we burn so each year we add a few pounds. The U.S. government says that by the year 2030, 50% of the U.S. population will be obese.

Getting fit is a comprehensive program. It can be slow and gradual. Little improvements are best so they become part of our lifestyle and don't require suffering. We do not want to engage in practices that are too uncomfortable or our fitness program is not likely to last. We will hit one milestone and decide that is enough.

Fitness becomes a lifestyle. It can become an addiction. Progress builds enthusiasm. Once we see that setting a goal, developing some discipline, and using our will power to overcome obstacles, we have unlimited capacity to get more fit.

Each year the RAAM (Race Across America) race begins in Oceanside, CA and ends in Annapolis, Maryland, 3,000 miles away. How and why do these people enter this race? The answer to that is the same as how man made so much progress since being a caveman.

It is the human spirit which is a drive to discover who we are. It is the brain desiring growth to make us feel vital. It is the body needing movement to feel at its optimum. There is no part of us that doesn't scream for growth and progress except our often lazy mind.

What is it about who we are that when its time to lace up our tennis shoes for a walk or run our mind says we are too tired or it will be too uncomfortable. This is the main obstacle to our greatness and finding out who we are. Sometimes a risk makes us hesitant. We are afraid of failure. We are afraid of finding out that we are not what we think we should be.

Nothing overcomes these obstacles like the first step and then the next step. One step at a time. Pretty soon we are running and are on top of the world with pride and satisfaction. Then comes gratitude, joy, and peace. Knowing who we are and why we are here is our purpose.

Fitness can be part of who you are. It can be part of why you are here. Those who make a recreation central to their lives are filled with gratification. Surfers are out at 6 a.m. to get that fix before they begin their day. The same can be said of runners, bikers, walkers and swimmers.

It is so easy for this new-found discipline to spread to other parts of our lives. I have become a disciplined writer. It started with difficulty in expressing myself clearly in a few paragraphs even though I am a college graduate. It is not easy to express ourselves. There is always the fear of sounding stupid when we begin. It's like taking your clothes off at the beach. What will others say? It takes practice but more than that it takes consistent engagement.

Then it becomes like taking a shower. We just do it.

Chapter Eight

Starting an Aerobics Program

Personal trainers and health coaches start sedentary people with a short walking regimen. They start with 10 minutes and stretch it to 30 minutes a day five days a week for a total of 150 minutes a week. After that, participants are encouraged to walk an hour a day for a total of 300 minutes a week.

If a person can run, then beginning a running program is better. They can start with 10 minutes and progress in the same manner. A treadmill is a comparable cardio exercise. Swimming can begin with a few laps and progress. Biking is a great exercise in which most people can engage.

The next phase for all these exercises is adding intensity. A first method of adding intensity is speed. One can increase speed or add intervals. Short bursts of speed followed by the normal pace.

Interval intensity is increased with greater speed, longer duration, or less rest between intervals. In phases one and two of a standard aerobics program, participants are barely exceeding their ability to talk while exercising. In the third phase, participants are increasing speed up to 80% of capacity and conversation is no longer possible.

In the final phase four, participants are increasing speed up to 95%. This phase is for competitors who might need to sprint at the end of a race. Their workouts are generally just once a week with the rest of the week devoted to phase one and two levels of intensity.

Chapter Nine

Exercises Leading up to Weight Training

Health coaches and personal trainers will often begin new clients that have been sedentary or having not engaged in weight training with floor exercises first. They will do the same with clients that are obese and may not have exercised in many years.

The purpose of beginning with floor exercises is to test balance and posture while creating the proper form. People who have not exercised may have bodies that are out of alignment. Lifting weights with a body out of alignment can create injuries. This should make sense. If you are straining with one part of the body taking extra load, then an injury can result.

Simple balance and posture exercises might include squats and lunges. These are good tests as well as exercises to start building muscle, cardiovascular fitness, and posture. Learning good form is crucial in preventing injury. Everyone wants to enter the gym and leave without injury.

Other exercises will test core strength. A plank is a good test and begins building basic core strength that will be instrumental for advancement. Various exercises can test abdominal strength. The core is only part stomach muscles and includes the whole abdominal region front and back.

Sitting on the floor with feet in front and under a weight with hands across chest and then testing one's ability to lean back tests core strength. This can progress into sit ups. One should only drop until the shoulders touch the floor or mat. Jerking to an upright position with the head on the floor can result in injury and fails to isolate the correct muscles.

Chapter Ten

Beginning Machine Weight Training

Most health coaches and personal trainers will move a new student first to machines rather than free weights. Machines are designed to control movement. They will help develop the right form. Maintaining the correct form is important to prevent injury.

A good beginner program includes lots of reps with light weights. These begin conditioning the muscles. Muscles need to develop receptors for glucose. Muscles not exercised for a long time have no receptors and most of the glucose from carbohydrates has been passing muscles and going to fat.

As muscles learn to absorb glucose, they increase in stamina. As they are exercised, they will start utilizing protein to grow. When muscles can't find adequate glucose, they will use fat for fuel. We see here the beauty of weight training to burn fat. As muscles recover, they will also burn fat and muscle. Getting the right nutrition to prevent muscles from consuming themselves is important.

A good goal for beginners is to reach 25 repetitions in a set. Then the exerciser tries to complete three sets with adequate rest in between. Intensity is increased by adding weights, adding more sets, or resting less between sets. There is lots of variety in this routine.

Another good goal is to include ten exercises in a routine of one set each. When the exerciser can complete ten exercises, they can repeat them. Completing this circuit three times is a different version of doing three sets of one exercise before moving on.

On different days, different routines could be the plan for the day. At first, because muscle is not being strained, exercisers could engage five days a week. They will begin to strengthen muscle, build receptors for glucose, start burning fuel, and gain stamina.

It is possible that if a new exerciser has been sedentary, they may begin with one day a week and then build to two and then every other day. It is important to move at a pace that is safe and comfortable. It is important to exercise safely, but not let the mind tell you you are tired when you are not.

A good way to warm the body and burn more calories is to begin with 5 minutes on a treadmill and end with 5 to 10 minutes on a treadmill. This has advantages to add calorie burn and muscles seeking fat for fuel as they recover. Then follow with a small protein and carbohydrate snack to keep the muscles feeding on fat and not on muscle.

Chapter Eleven

Beginning Free-Weight Training

The advantage of having begun with a machine-weight training program is many of the exercises can be duplicated with free weights. Free weights can be barbells and dumb bells as well as cables. It is possible that cables were already introduced during the machine-weight training stage.

Beginners should begin barbell and dumbbell training with less weight than they were using with machines. The benefits of barbell and dumbbell training is they add the need for balance. This requires more muscles to react. It is good to go lighter until such time as you can balance the weights properly.

Form is extremely important when moving to free weights. The machines are no longer guiding your movement. Now you could move in an improper manner which could minimize benefits or cause injury. Don't always learn by watching others at the gym. Better to have a trainer or watch YouTube videos which demonstrate proper form.

Barbells can be used on a machine and then dumbbells could be used for free weights. Executing squats, deadlifts, and various bench presses is still easier on the machine and less likely to result in injury.

Nonetheless, you still need proper form for exercises like squats or deadlifts or you could hurt your back. I once popped a vertebrae from improper squat form. My chiropractor popped it back in, but warned me about the dangers of improper form with squats. I since have made them my favorite exercise.

Dumbbells are on a rack and the exerciser uses the benches to assist in performing a wide variety of exercises. There are standing exercises like curls and reverse curls and lying down exercises like chest presses.

Once again, the exerciser might pick a routine of ten exercises and either execute three sets with light weights and 25 reps or do one after another with only one set. In performing 25 reps, the exerciser is lifting a weight that might be 25% to 40% of their one lift capacity. The one lift capacity will be a guess at the beginning.

If the exerciser is doing a routine of ten exercises with one lift per set, the set might include 25 reps with the lighter weight. At the end, the exerciser could do one or two more rounds. Exercising an hour five days a week is a goal once conditioning has improved. Muscles are not as greatly tested with lighter weights, so recovery is easier.

Chapter Twelve

Progressing to Heavier Weights

The next steps build different types of muscle. There are three types of muscle fibers and each is built with the three routines of light weights high reps, medium weight with 12 to 16 reps, and heavy weights with 5 to 8 reps.

As the weights get heavier, the exerciser is getting closer to their one lift capacity. True size and strength are not built until the third phase. In the medium or second phase the exerciser is lifting at 40% to 60% of one lift capacity. The sets of 12 to 16 reps is the right number to stress these muscle fibers. The idea is to tear them and allow them to build stronger.

As the exerciser progresses, he may notice that he is losing fat (inches) but not as much weight. Muscle is heavier than fat. In the first two phases, the exerciser should be burning fat as the muscles will seek fat for fuel and in recovery.

It is important to provide the right nutrients, but to cut out empty calories that add too many carbohydrates or bad fat. Sugar and flour should be the first nutrients to limit. Then eliminate high sodium foods that are in packages or consumed at restaurants. Bad oils are utilized by restaurants for fried and cooked foods.

In the second phase, the exerciser is lifting heavier weights and executing 12 to 16 reps. These should test one's upper limits. When they become too easy, it is a sign you could move to a heavier weight. Intensity can be increased with heavier weights, more sets, and less rest between sets.

In the third phase, the exerciser approaches maximum lift capacity. He should begin with 60% to 80% of one lift capacity in 5 to 8 reps. Three sets is a good goal. Once again, intensity is increased with heavier weights, more sets, and less rest between sets.

The exerciser might end his sessions with an attempt to lift his maximum weight up to 5 reps. This results in additional tearing and optimum rebuilding for size and strength. This should not be indulged more than once a week. After this routine, longer rest might be required. Muscle builds while resting. It might require two to four days to rest after extremely heavy lifting near maximum lift capacity. Overtraining can result in injury.

Exercisers using heavy weights to build their physique and appearance might still want to lose fat. They resort to all types of supplements. This requires caution. They also might engage in intermittent fasting which is eating in smaller windows during the day and allowing more time for the body to digest and utilize fat for fuel.

Chapter Thirteen

Beginning Cardiovascular Fitness

Aerobics increase the blood vessels in your body that transfer nutrients and eliminate wastes. Aerobics help build lung capacity and heart strength. Aerobics build stamina to increase the duration of exercises and speed recovery.

The sedentary person can begin slowly and will be amazed at how quickly they can progress. Patience and consistency are important. Discipline and willpower are important. There are days when your mind will say you don't want to walk or exercise. These are the days you must override your mind for you to make progress. Think of your goals and picture the new you.

Begin with a program that might be walking ten minutes a day 5 days a week. Progress to 30 minutes a day and then 60 minutes a day. At this point you would be exercising 300 minutes a week or 5 hours. This supports a weight loss program because the body begins to burn fat after it has used up its minimum supply of glucose (carbohydrates).

Swimming, biking, treadmills, and hiking all support building your cardiovascular system. Weight training complements your aerobic weight loss program by burning more calories and also consuming fat for fuel. Aerobics only can cause the body to burn your muscle for fuel.

Beginning cardiovascular exercises or aerobics start at a pace where you can exercise and talk comfortably. This is a measure of the amount of oxygen you are burning. Consistent exercise builds the body's ability to supply oxygen to the muscles. Increasing duration will begin the body's consumption of fat for fuel as carbohydrates are burned.

Surfing is an exercise that assimilates intervals. Paddling for waves burns oxygen quickly and muscles need glucose for energy and stamina. Then muscles need to recover quickly for the next round. They will utilize the nutrients stored and then they will begin burning fat for fuel. Training the body to burn fat with long slow aerobic sessions helps the body burn fat more quickly when fuel is needed.

Many people will find that minimum aerobics fits their needs and will be satisfied with a half hour walk or other exercise a day. It is a good start for getting into surfing shape. If you want to increase your stamina and the length of your surfing sessions, you may want to progress to more demanding aerobic exercising.

Chapter Fourteen

Advanced Cardiovascular Fitness

The next step in building an aerobics program can be exercising so that talking while exercising becomes more difficult. This means speeding up the pace. Increasing duration is also progress. Finally, introducing intervals is the phase used from intermediate to professional exercisers.

Increasing the pace of aerobics builds greater cardiovascular abilities. Introducing intervals in which you speed up and then slow down is considered the optimum aerobic conditioning and fat burning phase.

Intervals can be short such as one minute with a minute or two at the normal pace. Then interval times can be increased and still maintain the normal pace as rest.

To increase the intensity of intervals there are several alternatives. The speed can be increased. The duration can be lengthened. The rest can be shortened or any combination. At the same time, the duration of the entire exercise can be lengthened and the normal pace can be increased.

The reason athletes engage in intervals is they find that in addition to building capacity, their average speed increases. I ran 60 miles a week with a track club in my 30's and we trained weekly with intervals to increase average speeds for races. Most of our training was at our comfortable pace and then at least weekly we would push training to near capacity interval speeds.

Phase two of aerobics training is exercising at levels where talking is comfortable. Then the exerciser introduces intervals for growth. In this phase the exerciser might also speed up their pace to make talking and breathing more difficult. This training should be enough for people who want to run 10K's.

Phase three of aerobics training is exercising at high levels of intensity so talking and breathing are difficult. Intervals become more intense with increased speed, duration, and less rest between intervals. This becomes training for more intense events like longer races.

Phase four of aerobics training is for serious our professional athletes. These exercisers are racers and might need near capacity speed at the end of races. This phase includes normal paced training during the week with more intense intervals once a week.

If your goal is surfing, you are greatly increasing your ability to exercise longer and engage in more challenges like riding bigger waves. Paddling out further requires more confidence, endurance, and confidence in your stamina.

Chapter Fifteen

Building Flexibility

Flexibility in surfing is crucial. Professionals can wrap their legs around their necks in a sitting position like yogis. Flexibility is more than stretching. It is building the muscles involved in movement to strength so they can operate smoothly.

I like to stretch but can build flexibility without it. I build flexibility with three main exercises. I do burpies each morning. I do deadlifts with a 35 pound barbell plate. I do squats with the same plate.

When I get to the beach, I practice a few pop ups on the surfboard before I teach. I find my pop ups are strong and smooth. To test my flexibility, I put my palms flat on the ground without bending my knees. I achieve it, but the first exercises get me there better than stretching.

Upper body and core strength are also important in doing surfing pop ups and achieving flexibility. I do push ups and planks. Now I have built my upper body for pop ups and core strength for the pop to my feet.

These few exercises would complement almost any recreational exercise. The deadlifts and squats build leg strength while adding flexibility to the hamstrings, buttocks, and lower back.

You will find that everyday chores such as picking things up and lifting become much easier. You will also realize you don't worry about throwing out your back each time you have a chore or pick up something from the floor.

To go beyond surfing exercises, you could do yoga or pilates. These are spiritual and physical endeavors that broaden your capabilities and improve your lifestyle. Using cables can strengthen and stretch your muscles. A simple set of bands that wrap around a post or that you step on and pull can add lots of benefits.

A test of flexibility in beginning surfing is whether you can do the push up on the surfboard and then put your foot flat on the board under your butt. From here you rise as you move your other foot to the nose. Try this on your living room floor. Can you put your foot flat on the floor under your butt and stand on it?

Chapter Sixteen

Nutrition for Exercise and Weight Loss

Most people get in a habit of eating the same things every day. They also have their addictions. It is often the addictions that cause our weight gain. Our psychological need for something that is bad for us can add a few pounds every month.

I was always addicted to ice cream after dinner. Every time I wanted to lose weight, I began by ending this addiction. The best way I discovered was to substitute something that might also be bad. I might start having a Snickers Bar. Then after a week, I had broken the ice cream addiction, I moved to a granola bar. This worked every time.

Then, I would pinpoint other items in my diet that should be eliminated. I would focus on sugar and flour. These are the two most difficult items to eliminate for most people. It eliminates sweets, pasta, pizza, bread, cereal, desserts, sodas, sugary drinks, and pastries.

Next is bad cooking oils. This eliminates most restaurant and fast foods. This eliminates most packaged goods hidden in sweeteners and lots of sodium.

Lynn Genet-Recitas has a great weight loss book called *The Plan*. Working with thousands of clients she has found that everyone has food allergies and they are different. A food allergy causes inflammation. Inflammation causes weight gain. Elimination of foods that cause inflammation plus drinking lots of water results in weight loss.

Her plan begins with three days of basic foods she has found causes no inflammation in most people. After three days, you begin adding one food a day. If you lose at least a half pound a day, you were not allergic to the new food and are drinking enough water. If you gained weight, the item you added caused inflammation or you were not drinking enough water.

I lost 17 pounds in three weeks. I was also exercising seriously with lots of aerobics. My diet after four years of taking out bad foods and adding good foods had been reduced to a basic raw diet. I live that way today.

I have three meals with much less food than I used to eat. I find my body acclimates to this routine and I don't have the cravings or the up and down blood sugar crashes. I try to balance the protein, carbohydrates, and fat, but I lean on protein and fat.

My diet is basically a Keto diet with lots of protein and good fats with complementary fruits, vegetables, and nuts. This is not for everyone. It takes some conditioning. This diet is good for exercising. I am getting the basic essentials without nutrients that are empty calories (pastries).

Muscles need protein and glucose (carbohydrates) for fuel. When they are depleted of glucose, they will turn to fat for fuel. If they don't have the sufficient nutrition, they will also start eating the body's muscle. As we age, we can lose muscle as part of the aging process.

One of the problems of getting fit as a senior if we have been sedentary is we have lost muscle and strength. The muscles have to be constantly exercised or they atrophy. Exercised muscles have to be fed. As I have mentioned, when muscle is built, it has receptors for absorbing glucose in the blood. If muscle is not developed these receptors are gone and glucose goes to fat.

Building muscles, cardiovascular improvement, and flexibility toward fitness is a gradual process. Developing good nutrition is also a gradual process. Each requires patience, dedication, persistence, and will power. Ask yourself if your goals are worth it.

Chapter Seventeen

Catching Waves

The fun of surfing for beginners starts with catching waves. Many students who don't learn to stand up say they had great fun. Laying on a surfboard and feeling a foam wave start to push the board at 15 mph is exhilarating. Standing, of course, would be more fun, but just the feeling of being pushed by pure energy is a great reward. Waves are water energized by the wind.

Catching waves becomes the obsession of surfers for the rest of their lives. The better they become, the bigger waves they could ride. The second aspect is recognizing waves and how to catch them. Waves from day to day, low tide to high tide, and beach to beach are different.

The beginner surfer first learns how to roll over onto a surfboard as the foam wave is approaching and begins paddling to start the momentum. The surfer then looks back to see how close the foam wave is to the board. When the wave is only a few feet away, he paddles much harder in order to get in front of the wave.

The surfer does not want to remain with the tail of the surfboard in the foam as he tries to stand up. He wants to accelerate so the surfboard is being pushed by the little curved lip that is created as the foam waves moves to shore. This is where the smooth pop up and ride exist.

After the surfer learns how to catch the foam waves and ride to the beach, he can progress by paddling out through the waves and turning around to catch the next one. This begins to help surfers get comfortable in the ocean as they start selecting which waves to ride.

Paddling longer builds stamina quicker. Paddling is what makes surfers tired. This is the game. Paddle more to build stamina. It is like running. Start with a quarter mile and build stamina until you can run a mile.

Correct paddling occurs by dropping the arm into the water up to the elbow so most of the power is generated by the forearm. Strokes should be short and close to the board. Surfers do not want to hand paddle. Strokes should also be even with both arms. Many have a tendency when they begin in foam waves to paddle harder with one arm causing the board to carve sideways into the wave and then get turned over.

A high-volume surfboard makes paddling easier but not necessarily easy. There is still lots of work involved. If a person wanted to make paddling their exercise program, they could burn a lot of calories, build muscle, gain balance on the surfboard, get more comfortable in the ocean and improve a basic surfing skill.

Chapter Eighteen

Standing up On the Surfboard

Standing up on the surfboard is a main objective in surfing. Two others are catching waves and then riding them. The process of catching waves and standing up is about timing and rhythm.

Whether foam waves or real waves, the surfer sees the wave and makes a judgement about position and timing. As a beginner, you see foam waves arriving and decide when to roll over to start paddling and catch the wave.

In catching the foam wave, the surfer begins by rolling over 20 feet before the wave arrives noticing how big, how fast, and if it is coming at an angle. Then he starts paddling to get some momentum. As the wave gets close, the surfer paddles hard as the wave hits the board and until he feels the surfboard take off in front of the wave.

Then the surfer places his hands on the surfboard next to his chest in a man's push up position. Then he pushes and places his back foot on the surfboard flat and under his butt. The foot placement is about two feet from the tail and in the middle of the surfboard. The surfer stands on the rear foot/leg as he brings up his hands and moves the other foot close to the nose of the board.

When standing in the correct posture, the front and rear foot need to be about shoulder width apart and the front foot has to be close enough to the nose to hold it down but not so close the foot pushes the nose under water.

The correct posture on the surfboard is with the weight equal on the front and rear leg with the torso upright. The hips and shoulders are square to the front and the hands in front where they can be seen. If the posture is correct, the surfboard will go straight and little work or balance is needed.

People think surfing is about balance, but I have seen very few people who did not have adequate balance. The downfall is not executing the pop up properly and smoothly to arrive in the right posture. If the weight is not distributed correctly by having the weight equal on the right and left sides of the middle stringer of the surfboard, balance will not help much.

I have students practice this pop up on their living room floor. If you want to test your mettle, try it in your living room. It might be a window into your ability and the work you have to do to get in surf shape.

Chapter Nineteen

Lean is an Advantage for Surfing

Surfing requires upper body strength, leg strength, core strength, and stamina. People that put-on weight are often not exercising. In learning to surf, this is more of a problem than weight because there are lots of overweight surfers.

Surfing is a lot easier if a surfer is lean. There is the power to weight ratio which means the power to lift one's body off the surfboard. This would mean that regardless of the weight, if a surfer is strong enough, they can get their body into a standing position on the surfboard. I recently had a strong surfing student who was 260 pounds and did a nice job of riding the surfboard.

The upper body pushes the body off the surfboard to begin the pop up. But upper body strength is also needed to paddle. When a surfer gets tired paddling, the fatigue seeps through their body and they begin to falter in all areas.

Leg strength is needed to stand up on the surfboard. In the beginner pop up, the surfer has to stand up on their rear leg. This means that while in a lying down position, the surfer puts their rear foot on the board and lifts their entire weight up as they move the other foot to the front of the surfboard.

This is where flexibility is also crucial. The rear foot when placed on the surfboard must be placed under the butt and flat on the board. If a person is not well stretched, they cannot get their foot flat. If their foot is not flat, they cannot stand on it. Try touching the floor without bending your knees. This is a first indication of your flexibility. Putting your palms on the floor is better.

As mentioned earlier, flexibility is needed in the hamstrings, buttocks, and lower back. All three get tight in sedentary behavior. When a person is capable of exercise, the best two exercises for loosening these three areas are burpies and squats. Both can be engaged without weights. The burpies require cardiovascular fitness, so be careful.

Upper body strength is developed with pushups, bench presses, and cable pulls. They work together to give the strength to push off the surfboard and to paddle. Of course, nothing works for paddling like getting in the ocean and paddling or swimming. Swimming can be enjoyed anywhere without the need for the ocean and it is great cardiovascular training.

The process of standing up on the surfboard begins with catching the wave. Then the surfer places his hands on the surfboard in a man's push up position next to the chest. The surfer pushes up and puts their rear (right foot for most people) on the surfboard flat. Flat is crucial. The foot is slightly turned to the right. When the front foot lands, it will also be turned at a 45 degree angle to the right.

Then the surfer stands on that rear foot, and raises his hands and body as he moves the other foot to the nose of the board. The finishing stance should have the feet about shoulder width apart (3'). The hips and shoulders should be square to the front with both hands in front. Knees are flexed and weight is equal on front and back legs.

At this point the surfer is riding balanced to the beach. If the posture is correct, the surfboard will travel straight with very little work required to stay on the surfboard. If the posture is not correct, the surfer struggles to stay on the surfboard.

Chapter Twenty

Selecting the Right Surfboard

Beginners want to select a surfboard with a lot of volume to make learning to surf easier and also allow them to advance until such a time they may want to surf a shorter soft top board or purchase a hard board. Volume is calculated by multiplying length, times width, times thickness. There is a chart at the end of the book that matches weight with the volume of surfboard that should be purchased.

Beginners should start with high volume boards and move slowly in buying boards with less volume. Surfing progress is usually slow and moving to an advanced board can lead to more frustration than fun.

A beginner wants more volume for four reasons. They are easier to paddle. They catch foam waves easier. They are easier for doing the pop up. They are easier to ride. If any one of these gets more difficult, the fun drains out of the experience.

The beginner surfer begins near the shore rolling over onto the surfboard to catch foam waves and rides to the beach. The surfer then progresses to paddling out to ride bigger foam waves and starts catching small real waves. The soft top high-volume surfboard is great for this practice. The surfer should keep progressing trying to catch bigger real waves.

At this point, the beginner is now an intermediate surfer. On real waves, he will learn to drop down a small face. Then he will learn to angle the surfboard toward the pocket to prevent pearling (where the nose goes under water) before popping up. He may also learn bottom turns, cut- backs, and accelerating.

Now, he may decide he would like a hard board to improve maneuverability. The main advantage of a hard board over a soft top is that the rails are thinner to allow the surfer to dig the rail into the wave for sharper carves. Up to this point, there is no need to jump to a hard board.

The progress to shorter hard boards from soft tops should be very gradual. The surfer should buy boards just 6 inches shorter at a time trying to maintain good width and thickness. As soon as the volume drops, the paddling is more difficult, catching waves requires more advanced timing, popping up is more unstable, and riding is more unstable.

One way to progress is to move to lower volume soft tops. I often start surfers on a 9' soft top and move them to an 8' soft top. An 8' soft top is a great board and could last a surfer all their life, especially if they don't get in the ocean often. I still ride an 8' soft top and lots of surfers in the line up are riding them. You can ride 7' high waves with them. I also have short boards.

Overweight surfers want at least a 9-foot soft top surfboard. Surfers over 200 pounds would be better served by soft tops that are at least 24 inches wide and near three inches thick. This should suffice up to about 260 pounds. After that, a beginner should consider Stand Up Paddle (SUP) boards. A 9'6" SUP can be 33 inches wide and over 4 inches thick.

Start with the appropriate high-volume surfboard as you begin to lose weight. As a surfer loses weight, they can consider progressing to lower volume soft tops. There are also high-volume hard boards. Hard boards are available up to 12 feet long and have big widths and thickness.

I think a good-sized hard board if a surfer doesn't want to go shorter are boards that are 9' or 9'6". Width and thickness can be varied for better flotation. These boards have lots of volume and are still maneuverable. Lots of surfers are on these boards and the long board surfer has a certain style that usually has them gathering together on beaches where the waves favor long boards. This is usually a reef where the waves form slowly and have nice shape. Sand bar bottom beaches don't allow the waves to form as slowly and often have what are called "close out" waves. These waves are steep and can cause long boards to pearl more easily.

Chapter Twenty-One

Choosing a Wetsuit

Wetsuits make surfing comfortable when the water is colder than you personally would enjoy in your swim trunks. Everyone has different tolerances. On days when some people are wearing thick wetsuits, others are in their swim trunks with a rash guard.

Generally, there are three seasons of water temperatures. I have three different weight wetsuits because I am in the water all year. For the winter, I have a thick full wetsuit with a thickness called 4/3. This means the chest and back area have a layer that is 4 mm and the arms and legs have a layer that is 3 mm. The thicker layer keeps the core organs warmer.

This wetsuit is great for the winter when water temperatures in Oceanside drop into the 50's. More important for me because I am standing when I teach is resilience to the ocean breezes. For me, they are what make me get cold when I am in the water a few hours.

In the spring and fall when water temperatures are a little warmer, I have a full wetsuit that is the 3/2 thickness. In the summer when the water temperatures are above 70, I have a summer suit that has short sleeved arms and legs.

Wetsuits come in various qualities. My winter suit has a graphene lining which I find is terrific for both cold and wind. In general terms, a full 4/3 winter wet suit can run from $160 to $500. Depending on your country and water temperatures, different qualities may be necessary.

Sizes vary greatly. Each manufacturer has a chart on their website and they are based on weight and height. In my last research, wetsuits seem to top out at 3xxx large which is suitable up to 260 pounds. If you are larger, you might have to do more research to find a wetsuit.

Chapter Twenty-One

Learn to Surf and Change Your Life

When beginning on a venture it is good to have a worthwhile goal. A person beginning a nutrition and exercise program would be more motivated when he has an ambitious goal. He knows the challenge it will create and how fit he will have to be in order to be successful.

Navy Seals face some of the most rigorous training possible, but they know passing the tests are necessary to become a Seal. Only a few percent of the best qualified military personnel can pass the test. That alone is a badge of honor.

They are training to face the unknown. They may be training to accomplish extremely difficult or impossible missions. They may be facing another country's best military personnel or overwhelming obstacles. Landing in Pakistan a few miles from a military base to find Bin Laden was a daring task.

In face of these facts, learning to surf shouldn't be as difficult. It is not life threatening. In fact, it might be life-saving. Thinking of people accomplishing something more difficult than what you are trying to do might be encouragement that you can do it.

Everyone facing a challenge needs a good goal, discipline, focus, and resilience. In his book, "Resilience", Navy Seal and Rhodes scholar Eric Greitens said Seal Training is the greatest experience you never want to repeat. You learn how to face challenges you're not sure you can accomplish. What could be more fun than that?

One can wonder what goes through the mind of people like Elon Musk who keep doing what others would think is impossible. He took on the automotive industry with an electric car. He took on NASA by developing his own rocket ships. He built batteries big enough to bolster Australia's electric grid. Doesn't he ever worry about failure? Of course, he does.

One of the elements of surfing, I tell my students, is that fear is the 800-pound gorilla in the room. Most people have a little fear of the ocean's power. A wave is about speed and weight. It can weigh thousands of pounds when it falls on you if it is a big wave. One learns quickly that the power of waves is greater than a person's ability to withstand them without technique.

Champion big wave surfers said they were afraid each time they started surfing the next bigger sized waves. On real big days at Teahupoo, a big wave in Tahiti, recently, the surfers said they were even terrified, but this was their profession and what they chose in life.

A challenge might not be worthwhile if it doesn't scare you a little bit. It might not be worth your best efforts if there isn't a chance of failure. Doing what we know we can do is often boring. Doing work that is not challenging is stifling. Not growing is not your purpose.

The brain needs challenge to stay vital. Without challenge, it begins to decline. The end point of a declining brain is dementia; it's just a matter of time.

We can learn all our lives because our brains have plasticity. Whenever you focus on something difficult that is a challenge, your brain grows. It is important to keep your brain growing.

Nothing the brain loves more than learning something physical. Learning how to walk as youngsters is one of the brains greatest challenges in life. Learning language is a second great feat. The brain grows enormously during these periods. After that we often stop testing the brain to the same degree.

If you are going to get healthy and fit so you can learn to surf, you are going to have lots of challenges. You are going to have to learn how to overcome obstacles. The biggest obstacle will be fighting your own willpower. You will have to make changes your mind will tell you are not good for you, at first.

The beauty of progressing is that soon your mind signs on to the mission and is your greatest fan. Exercise can become addicting. Someone starts off jogging, or weightlifting, or getting thinner and pretty soon they are addicted. The brain loves health and fitness.

Let's get started!

Bibliography

Mark Kaplan

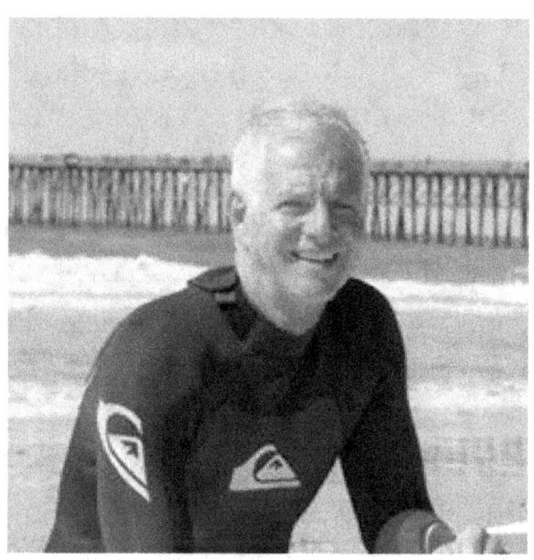

I have been a life-long enthusiast of exercise
and health. Most sports and recreation have
been attractive to me and I have tried as many
as possible. My love was running and I started
jogging in high school and running more
seriously with a community track club as an
adult.

Surfing was a high school adventure but became more of an addiction after I retired. Daily surfing and website building for others led to a surfing website which became highly rated by Google for surf lessons in Oceanside. This became my accidental backing into the business of teaching surf lessons.

Noticing how many of my students from kids to seniors were overweight and not in good condition led me to a certification by Ace as a Health Coach. I also pursued courses in Personal Training and Nutrition.

Surfing is just one great goal for motivating a change in one's personal fitness. Pursuing health and fitness is a lifestyle and affords many benefits. I hope this book leads to your desire to make lifestyle changes.

www.ingramcontent.com/pod-product-compliance
Lightning Source LLC
Chambersburg PA
CBHW061525250726
48657CB00005B/2090